Kelly Wislar

Have-A-Seat Yoga™

Have-A-Seat Yoga™ :

Inspiration to Get Started, Stay Connected, and Keep Going

by
Kelly Wislar and Susan Marg

Breath To Balance Media   *   San Diego   *   2019

MILL CITY PRESS

Mill City Press, Inc.
2301 Lucien Way #415
Maitland, FL 32751
407.339.4217
www.millcitypress.net

© 2019 by Kelly Wislar and Susan Marg

First Edition
A Book for Inspiration
Published by Breath to Balance Media

All images by Anatolir/Shutterstock.com

Printed in the United States of America

LCCN: 2019920439
ISBN-13: 978-1-5456-8082-7

With heartfelt gratitude
to my family and friends.
– Kelly Wislar

To my husband James C. Simmons,
for enriching my life with his love and
inspiration.
– Susan Marg

TABLE OF CONTENTS

Read a Book

Practice Mindfulness

Talk the Talk

Live the Life

Help for the Common Cold

Help for Back Pain

Help for Osteoarthritis

Help for Insomnia

Help for Fatigue

Help for Headaches

Help for Diabetes

Help for Indigestion

Help for Memory Loss

Help for Heart Disease

ACKNOWLEDGEMENTS

Most importantly, I would like to thank one of my original students, James C Simmons, who suggested I write a book based on my program to target a population that is often overlooked. On his recommendation, I met and collaborated with his wife Susan, who has since become a good friend. Over the next eighteen months we produced a book that is meant to unite people, as well as motivate them to try something new.

I would also like to thank my yoga instructor, Katie Brauer, for inspiring me. She generously gave me the seed that I planted, and it has grown into something much bigger than I could have ever imagined.

My heart goes out to my family and RSC. They give me strength and purpose to live each day in love and light.

Namaste,

Kelly Wislar

INTRODUCTION

Inspiration is the influence on the mind or emotions to be, to learn, to create. It comes from deep inside us or from places or people far away. The word itself is derived from the Latin meaning to draw breath into the lungs, a basic principle of yoga when done deeply with concentration.

I took up yoga when I was forty years old to recover from cancer and discovered its healing power. After becoming a certified yoga instructor, I began to teach in assisted living facilities. Some of my students were in wheelchairs. Almost everyone else moved with difficulty, Today, I get my inspiration from them, the young at heart with the will to keep going.

One of my first students, a 96-year-old gentleman, felt wonderful learning something new and expanding his horizons, something that connected him to his daughter, a yoga practitioner herself, as well as the outside world. Another student, a woman in her eighties still living independently, was delighted to realize that she had improved her tennis game because of the stretches and twists incorporated into each session. Several of those I teach have been pursing yoga for decades and don't want to give it up despite getting older. I give private lessons to my neighbor, a retired NFL player, who is intent on staying alert and mobile.

I adapted a general yoga routine to Have-A-Seat Yoga™, so everyone can participate. Even if you can no longer get down on the mat or up from the floor, you can achieve the many physical, psychological, and social benefits of yoga with practice. This book has ten chapters with ten topics per chapter. It addresses the questions you might have about Have-A-Seat Yoga™, such as what to wear and how often to practice, and it includes suggestions on how to overcome your fears, reduce stress, and bring balance into your life. If you are not convinced that this is for you, medical school-conducted research that documents the value of yoga, from controlling your blood pressure and relieving aches and pains to sleeping better through the night, is summarized in the last chapter.

For more inspiration, each topic concludes with a Sanskrit word associated with yoga or a quote from a contemporary or historical artist, actor, scientist, political leader, or business person, among others. Here's one of my favorites:

"If you change the way you look at things, the things you look at change."– Wayne Dyer

Here's another:

**What an elder sees sitting; the young can't see standing."
– Gustave Flaubert**

Yoga is a process which you are never too old to begin. It encompasses the concepts of mindfulness, gratitude, and connection, as well as the physical postures that so many of us associate with yoga. Have-A-Seat Yoga™ is fun, safe, and doable. It's time to get started.

Namaste,

Kelly Wislar

Chapter 1

GETTING STARTED

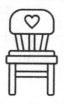

What Am I Getting Into?

Yoga is not about skinny women wearing leotards or twisting yourself into a pretzel. Rather, it is a set of exercises or positions along with meditation that restores or strengthens the mind and body connection, so you are stronger and more flexible, free from stress.

Have-A-Seat Yoga™ is the same, although you don't have to get down on the floor and get up from your mat. As the term suggests, it is practiced in a chair. If you are up to it, you can twist, stretch, bend forward and even backwards while sitting. When performed on a regular basis, you will achieve all the health benefits, both physical and psychological, of yoga.

It's perfect for seniors who can't get around like they used to or who want to hold on to what they have. Children, too, can practice chair yoga at their desks, possibly before a presentation or a big test, or with their family, just to have fun. Desk-bound workers can let go of the tensions of the day right where they're at. It's really for everyone.

Try it. Put a stretch in your hands. Extend your fingers. Exhale. Make a tight fist and squeeze. Touch those shoulders. Bring your elbows together. Now repeat.

The Sanskrit word 'yoga' means connection. The practice of yoga is the union of body, mind, and spirit.

No Artificial Flavors

Everything in yoga comes from nature. Many of the names of yoga postures are based on objects of beauty and strength that we find all around us. While I haven't translated all of the yoga positions mentioned below into chair yoga, the relationship between yoga and nature can be seen.

The lotus flower deserves special mention as it has been a symbol in Eastern religion for thousands of years. It represents being fully grounded in murky ponds and muddy streams while growing towards the light.

The butterfly pose imitates a butterfly resting its wings on a lotus blossom. To get into the pose you bring the soles of your feet together while sitting on the floor. If practicing from a chair, you can meditate on the beauty of this image.

There are other poses, too, such as the eagle, a god in Indian mythology, and the cobra, a reptile that is sacred and revered in India. Our best friend is appreciated by the upward and downward facing dog. Mountains and trees evoke strength, and the poses carrying their names improve balance.

Yoga also pays tribute to the moon and the sun. What can be more inspiring than rising with the sun and saying goodnight to the silvery satellite in our earthly sky? We honor these celestial objects with salutations comprised of a series of postures which we coordinate with our breathing. A sun salutation warms the body and stimulates the soul. A moon salutation cools the body and quiets the mind.

"Study nature, love nature, stay close to nature. It will never fail you." – Frank Lloyd Wright

Take a Breath

Breathing is fundamental to life, and it is the basis of yoga. It moves energy through the body and gets the body moving. To fill their hearts with life at the start of every session that I teach, I instruct my students to think of something that brings them joy. I suggest that they remember a person whom they miss, a trip which they took, or a book that they read. I tell one of my students, a retired writer, to think of one of his books. This always makes him smile.

Throughout the session, I continuously remind students to breathe. "Breathe life into your heart," I tell them. "Remember to breathe." You never want to hold your breath.

The Sanskrit word "prana" means life force. It is the energy that keeps us vibrant and animated. It is also used to refer to breath.

Make a Roadmap

GPS is not needed. Decide where you want to go and set goals. Put yourself on the right path to get there, and Have-A-Seat Yoga™ is a step in the right direction. With chair yoga your body will become more flexible, and your mind will follow, free from stress. It's not easy, but anything worthwhile never is.

Many practitioners begin yoga for healing, physical healing after an accident or an illness. Emotional, as well as spiritual healing, is often the next step. My personal journey began when I had cancer when I was forty years old. I don't want to be too dramatic, but yoga saved me. Developing and teaching Have-A-Seat Yoga™ has made me one with the universe.

> **"You have brains in your head. You have feet in your shoes. You can steer yourself any direction you choose." – Dr. Seuss**

See Yourself Succeeding

Basketball players see themselves making the shot. Corporate leaders picture themselves giving a rousing presentation. And they accomplish their goals.

Now, what about you? You haven't played basketball since your youngest son left for college and you have never given a formal presentation to a large audience, nor do you want to. Still, there are situations in which you find yourself where visualization can help you succeed.

Imagine yourself doing yoga, sitting in a chair, breathing deeply, stretching fully. Envision the many benefits you will receive, from sleeping better to standing taller.

Visualize getting up from a chair without assistance or waiting patiently for your ride who is always late. Think about preparing dinner without snacking or getting dressed without help.

You, too, can utilize the power inside you to improve your performance, not just during a practice, but in your everyday life.

"If you can dream it, you can do it." – Walt Disney

Take a Class. Buy a Book. Watch a Video.

If you want to start doing chair yoga, many senior housing communities and assisted living facilities now offer instruction as part of their scheduled activities. Yoga studios and community centers also offer classes, and they have become as ubiquitous as your favorite coffee shop.

In a class, you get encouragement and assistance from your instructor. He or she checks to see if you are doing a posture correctly, so you don't hurt yourself.

Classes also come with a social benefit. You are not alone. You might have different goals than your fellow practitioners, but you also have something in common with them. During a session, you produce energy, and your energy is compounded by that of others in your class. Your journey, wherever you want to go, becomes a step easier.

If you're a self-starter or you can't easily get to a class, buy a book, check out YouTube, or watch a video. There are now bookshelves filled on the topic and videos that can be streamed or watched on a DVD player. And you can get started in your practice in the comfort of your home.

> **"I am always doing that which
> I cannot do, in order that
> I may learn how to do it."**
> **– Pablo Picasso**

Get Dressed

While clothes might make the man or woman, they make no difference when you practice yoga. Sure, you can put on Lululemon leggings or a pair of bright pink or blue sweatpants with matching shirt, but no one cares how you look. If you are taking a class, you might imagine that your instructor is looking at you funny, especially if you're dressed for the golf course, but he or she is most likely only checking to see if you're doing the exercises correctly or whether you need some assistance.

Still, it is recommended that you wear loose fitting clothing for chair yoga. A baggy pair of old jeans will be just fine, but they should be worn in and stretched out. You don't want to feel confined or constrained because that impacts the way you move. For your practice you want to be able to move freely. Just remember that everyone is a critic, so if you wear plaids with polka dots, someone is going to complain.

Shoes or no shoes, it's up to you. It is common practice to be barefoot in a yoga

studio, so you can grip the floor for balance.
Have-A-Seat Yoga™ is another matter. Make
yourself comfortable. Make yourself at home.

**"Age and size are only numbers.
It's the attitude you bring
to clothes that make the
difference." – Donna Karan**

Pull Up a Chair

For Have-A-Seat Yoga™ , any chair will do, although some are more appropriate than others. Perhaps you'll choose a chair from the dining room or the kitchen. The chair in which you sit to watch TV might be too soft. The best chair is one that is firm and armless, so you can raise your arms out to the side during some of the poses. A fold up chair is great, if you want to change rooms or move outside. Still, you want to be careful to limit your distractions, if you are easily distracted by bees and flowers.

I also have classes where many of the practitioners are in wheelchairs. Wheelchairs are always welcome.

> **"What an elder sees sitting;**
> **the young can't see standing."**
> **– Gustave Flaubert**

Do Something for Yourself

You deserve to be happy and fulfilled. You've worked hard to raise a family, but you still worry about your children and now their children. You have money in the bank, but you are concerned that it won't be enough. You have scrapbooks of happy pictures of places you've been, but you can't travel anymore, although you would love to go on a trip.

What now? It's time to do something for yourself. Have-A-Seat Yoga™ will put a smile on your face and love in your heart.

> **"What lies behind us and what lies before us are tiny matters compared to what lies within us." – Ralph Waldo Emerson**

Smile

Smile because it's a beautiful day, even if it is raining. Smile because the world will smile with you. Smile because you are trying something new. Smile before you begin your practice. Smile during your practice. Smile after your practice. It's all good.

"Smile in the mirror. Do that every morning and you'll start to see a big difference in your life." – Yoko Ono

Chapter 2

FROM THE BEGINNING

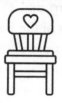

Back to the Future

Yoga has been pursued for thousands of years. It has connections to Hinduism and Buddhism, but its practice in the West is generally not religious. In the very late 19th and early 20th centuries, yoga masters came West, and the practice began to catch on. In 1947, its popularity increased with the opening of a studio in Hollywood, California. In 1968, the Beatles went to India to study meditation and made headlines around the world, creating even more interest in the Eastern philosophy.

In 2016, it was estimated that there were over thirty-six million yoga practitioners in the United States who spent almost $17 billion on clothing, accessories, classes, and equipment, and the numbers are predicted to increase. Americans believe that yoga is good for them because it increases flexibility and strength, as well as relieves stress, among other benefits. There are studies that prove that this is true. Yoga's spiritual connotations are in the eye of the beholder or, in this case, the practitioner.

"The rhythm of the body, the
melody of the mind, and
the harmony of the soul
create the symphony of life."
– B.K.S. Iyengar

Find What Works for You

Many of the types of yoga that are followed today in Western culture, and there are many, were adapted from Hatha yoga, which emphasizes physical exercises or postures combined with breath training.

Athletes want a good, demanding workout, and power yoga, developed in the 1970s, is a good fit for them. From the school of Ashtanga yoga, it provides high-intensity training, and many of the postures focus on building strength and endurance. Hot yoga, originally practiced as Bikram yoga, is perfect for those who want to sweat. As the term implies, students practice under hot and steamy conditions, usually in rooms of 90 to 100 degrees Fahrenheit. Yin yoga is slow-paced, whereby beginning practitioners hold postures from forty-five seconds to two minutes. The more advanced hold out for five minutes or more.

Many might perceive goat yoga as nothing more than a passing fad. It might be, but we are not here to judge. The concept came to life on an Oregon farm where goats roamed freely.

When yoga classes were held, the goats joined in. They climbed the backs of the practitioners or provided warmth and comfort, allowing students to cuddle with them. It's an example of animal-assisted therapy, and many find it helps them cope with their problems.

Chair yoga has been around for some time, although it actually started as a tool to help practice certain postures, such as a forward bends. In that regard, it was similar to using blocks for height and support or straps to deepen stretches. As a type of yoga in and of itself, it is intended for seniors, who can no longer move easily, but it is also ideal for people of all ages with and without disabilities.

Some of my students have practiced yoga for ten, twenty, and even thirty years before joining me in Have-A-Seat Yoga™, not wanting to lose what they had gained.

**"Life is trying things to see if
they work." – Ray Bradbury**

Go with the Flow

Back in the sixties, do you remember anyone telling you to "go with the flow?" It's similar to "chill," but the opposite of "freaking out," "going ape," and "having a cow." The expression might be dated, but it's perfect for describing the flowing movement coordinated with the breath when transitioning from one posture to another in various styles of yoga.

In Vinyasa or Ashtanga yoga, for example, each pose is held, but you quickly assume the next pose. The idea is to move smoothly and swiftly through the series of exercises to get a good workout. Other derivatives of Hatha yoga are more deliberate, holding the postures themselves to improve concentration. Whatever style of yoga you practice, you don't want to go too fast or too slow. You want to move at a speed that's just right for you.

"Go with the flow" is a good motto by which to live your life and keep your blood pressure from rising. Hippies knew what they were talking about. Rock on.

"It does not matter how slowly you go as long as you do not stop." – Confucius

The Picture Perfect Pose

Get ready to start moving. The physical postures or poses, called asanas in Sanskrit, are illustrated in most books on yoga. Practicing various postures, the basis of any yoga session in Western culture, will give you control of your body, and control of your body gives you control of your mind.

Yes, yoga is exercise, but it is fun. With practice, you will stand taller and move more confidently. When you tie your breath to a posture, you will help your body work better, and you'll feel better, too. In Have-A-Seat Yoga™, we inhale when we raise our arms to the sky. We exhale when we lower them to our sides.

If you are a beginner, remember that no one is perfect, that no posture is executed perfectly. Ease of doing any given posture comes with time. You can hold your posture steady when your mind is steady. Do what you can. Yoga is not a competition. Get there when you can. Yoga is not a race.

"Perfection is attained by slow degrees; it requires the hand of time." – Voltaire

Pause

We breath when we walk. We breath when we talk. We breath all the time, and we don't even think about it.

However, in yoga, it is different. We think about our breathing, and we focus on inhaling, retaining, exhaling, retaining. We do breathing exercises to improve our concentration, to center on who we really are. Conscious breathing is a way to be present, to be in the here and now, rather than churning past events, be they successes or failures, in our mind. Conscious breathing is liberating. It takes us to a higher plane, one not driven by anxiety and self-doubt.

In my classes I focus on breathing. "Inhale," I tell my students, and then I count slowly to three and pause. "Exhale," I coach and then count slowly to three and pause. I repeat these instructions for about five minutes. It's so restful that some of my students fall asleep. I don't take it personally. It's not about me. It's about you, and it's important for you to be comfortable. Still, open your eyes if they get heavy, and soar.

The Sanskrit word "pranayama" means control of breath.

Mind Over Matter

Meditation, like conscious breathing, helps us focus. It makes us pause and listen, so we can figure out what is happening in our lives. It's an experience, and it plays a major role in a yoga practice.

Meditation begins with relaxation. You can meditate lying down or sitting up. If you are in a chair, sit away from the back of the chair with your feet firmly on the floor and aligned with your hips and knees. If you can, let your arms drop to your side or place your hands palms down on your lap. To generate heat and energy, place your right hand on top of the other with your thumbs touching. Relax your shoulders, back, and face muscles, and hear what you have to say.

The Sanskrit word "dhyana" means to contemplate or meditate.

Give Peace a Chance

There's no reason to be angry all the time. Peace comes from within. Meditating using a mantra is a positive way of relaxing the mind, so you feel cool, calm, and collected, at one with the world.

The most famous mantra in the world is "Om." On the most basic level, it is simply a sound, but it is a sound that resonates deep within the soul. You can feel the vibes when you take a deep breath and slowly release it as the sound travels into the universe. When practitioners in a class say it at the same time, there's harmony, and it is real.

Begin and end your practice reciting a mantra. This will help you separate the time you are spending on yourself from everything else you have to do for everyone else that day.

If you don't have a mantra, you can create your own. It can be as simple or complex as you want it to be. Choose any word that is meaningful to you, that you want to focus on, or simply focus on your breath.

If your mind wanders, so be it. It will come back.

The Sanskrit word "mantra" means mind instrument.

Strike a Happy Balance

Life is like a balance beam. One step just a little too far to the right, oops. Off you go. One step just little too far to the left, oops. Down you fall.

There are many yoga postures that help develop your balance. The most well-known involve standing up, such as the Tree. It is done with one foot resting on the opposite leg. Your arms are raised over your head with your palms together.

Oh, you are in chair. Oh, you can't raise your leg. Well, raise your arms and breathe deeply.

Balance is more than physical. It's mental, too. Have-A-Seat Yoga™ will help you create inner stillness, so you can balance life's demands.

> **"I always try to balance the light with the heavy–a few tears of human spirit in with the sequins and the fringes." – Bette Midler**

Take Charge

If it is difficult to concentrate while meditating, decide what you want to focus on during your practice. How do you want to help yourself? What stress do you want to eliminate? Then, with every cycle of breath, repeat your goals. Here are some examples:

Inhale good.
Exhale bad.

Inhale love.
Exhale hate.

Inhale calm.
Exhale stress.

Inhale fresh air.
Exhale stale air.

Inhale light.
Exhale darkness.

Inhale confidence.
Exhale doubt.

Now, create your own, and breathe.

**"Concentration is a fine antidote
to anxiety." — Jack Nicklaus**

Cool Down

At the end of your session, it is time to unwind and prepare yourself for getting back to your life. If you are able, there is a pose, called the "corpse pose" or "savasana", whereby you lie flat on the floor with your arms and legs spread out and your eyes closed. To go into this pose, begin by feeling that your body is sinking into the ground, and relax. It is at this time that healing of your body and your mind takes place.

If you are in a chair, you can also have this experience. You can close your eyes. You can roll your head from side to side. You can move your shoulders down and away from your ears. You can let go of your lower body and then your upper body, first by tensing and then releasing your muscles. You can listen to your breath. You can say your mantra. You can envision a warm light moving through your body.

And relax.

Take as much time as you need. When you are ready to come out of this pose, slowly become aware of your surroundings. Gradually awaken your toes and fingers and then the rest of your body.

Before ending the session, tell yourself to stay relaxed as long as possible. Say "namaste," and thank your teacher.

The Sanskrit word "namaste" means "I bow to you." It is a greeting of profound respect that is often accompanied by placing your hands together near your heart and bowing your head.

Chapter 3

BUILDING
YOUR PRACTICE

Try it. You'll like it.

This advertising slogan for Alka Seltzer entered our lexicon way back in 1972. In a television commercial, a diner at a steak house speaks directly to the television audience and tells them that his waiter suggested that he try a new menu item. After repeatedly being badgered to "Try it. You'll like it." he tried it. Not only didn't he like it, but it also gave him indigestion. Alka Seltzer cured his indigestion, and that he liked.

There was also a Life cereal commercial from the same time. Some kids are reluctant to try something new, so they have their little brother Mikey try it first. Guess what? Mikey liked it. And you will, too.

Once you have tried Have-A-Seat Yoga™, you have to keep going, if you want to change yourself and your world.

> **"If you change the way you look at things, the things you look at change." – Wayne Dyer**

Have No Fear

Are you afraid to try Have-A-Seat Yoga™ ? Why? Are you afraid of failure? Maybe, you are afraid of looking foolish when you try a new posture or you worry that you won't be able to meditate. Possibly, you are afraid that painful memories will surface when you meditate. Don't let fear keep you from success.

We all have courage to overcome our fears. It might be deep inside, but it's there. Whether or not you are aware of your courage, you use it every day. It takes courage to say "no" to your family when you need time alone. It takes courage to ask for a raise or a promotion when you deserve it. And it takes courage to try something new, to travel into unknown territory, even if that's where you want to go.

The Cowardly Lion didn't think he had courage, but that didn't keep him from going down the yellow brick road.

"Courage is what it takes to stand up and speak; courage is also what it takes to sit down and listen." – Winston Churchill

Start Small

As we get older, we don't move as fast as we once did. That's all right. There's no hurry. We have probably lost some of our flexibility, as well.

Trying to achieve a certain level of physical activity is a great goal for your Have-A-Seat Yoga™ practice, but you should be aware of what is happening to your body as you hold a posture or you move from one posture to another. Yoga should never create pain; it should relieve pain. If your breathing is uneven, slow down. If you are trying to do too much, and your body will tell you that this is so, stop. When you are ready, assume another posture carefully and gently.

It's important to understand what you can and can't do on any given day. Begin slowly, and you will improve. What is most important is to begin.

> **"Start where you are. Use what
> you have. Do what you can."**
> **– Arthur Ashe**

Own It

Make your practice your own. Yoga and chair yoga can become a lifelong pursuit. Gurus, who have been practicing yoga for many hours a day for many years on their personal path to enlightenment, have certainly made it so.

If you seek self-realization, a guru can provide assistance. If you want to improve your movements during practice, a yoga instructor can guide you. But how long you practice each day or how many times a week you pull up a chair is up to you.

The Sanskrit word "guru" means dispeller of darkness. A guru is a spiritual teacher.

Listen to Your Body

Only you know what you need to get through the day. A morning affirmation might be a part of your daily routine. "Nothing is going to bother me today," you might tell yourself as you greet the day. "I can deal with whatever challenges come my way," you might say as you reach for your bathrobe. Now, make it happen.

Practicing Have-A-Seat Yoga™ for a short period of time when you awake, and I recommend every morning, might be enough for you to get going and keep going. Many find that three minutes is enough to alleviate immediate concerns and create some energy, even before the first cup of coffee.

If you have a class that day, by all means go! You might not feel like it, but it will do you good.

> 'With the new day comes new
> strength and new thoughts."
> – *Eleanor Roosevelt*

Don't Kid Yourself

If a tree falls in a forest and no one is around to hear it, does it make a sound? If you only practice two to three times a year, are you really a practitioner? Whether the question is asked from a scientific or philosophical perspective, the answer depends on your perception, as well as your goals.

To do yourself some good, you need to practice two to three times a week. You want to challenge yourself, but not strain yourself. If you want to take a day off, take a day off. It's your practice, and there is no right or wrong. Still, I encourage everyone to be consistent, whether you are at home or taking a class.

**"The most effective way to do it,
is to do it." – Amelia Earhart**

Find Me Time

You think you don't have time to catch your breath, but you do. You think you don't have room on your calendar for one more activity, but you do. You think you don't have time to take a class, but you do.

Classes in Western culture focus not only on the postures, but on coordinating the postures with breath. You want to inhale when you raise arms and exhale when you lower your arms. It might feel awkward because usually you don't think about breathing.

Think about all the positive things that happen by breathing deeply and consciously when practicing yoga. Breathing keeps a steady supply of oxygen in the blood. Breathing links the body and the mind. Breathing reduces stress and gives you balance.

Yoga sessions typically last an hour, including time to acclimate at the start of class and then cool down when it's over. Classes don't last long enough to be an excuse not to attend.

See, you have the time.

"They always say time changes
things, but you actually have
to change them yourself."
– Andy Warhol

Drink Up

Unless you are lost at sea, having a glass of water is as simple as turning on the tap. This is a good thing. Water serves a plentitude of purposes. It helps control our body temperature, heart rate, and blood pressure. It's a thirst-quencher, too.

If you want something besides water, coffee counts towards our daily intake of fluid, as does a glass of juice. There's water in food, especially green vegetables, such as lettuce, celery and spinach, and juicy fruits, including watermelon, strawberries, and tomatoes. Yes, tomatoes are a fruit.

As with any exercise, you want to stay hydrated. If you don't, you might become dizzy or develop a headache. Have some water before practice. Take some sips during practice. Replenish yourself after practice.

"Water is the driving force of all nature." – Leonardo da Vinci

You Are What You Eat

Your body needs food. Your mind needs rest. Your soul needs balance. To take care of your body, mind, and soul you should eat well.

A yoga diet is based on whole grains, fresh fruits and vegetables, nuts and seeds, beans and legumes, and a moderate amount of dairy. You don't have to become a vegetarian to practice yoga but it has happened: some yogis become vegetarian. Some lose weight.

To aid digestion, eat slowly, enjoy every bite, and mind your p's and q's when you're at the dinner table. You will feel better and be healthier from the inside out. You'll also be good company for anyone joining you.

The Sanskrit word "mitahara" means the habit of moderate food.

Keep It Simple

Life can be complicated. Yoga needn't be.

Some yoga postures can be difficult, but they can also be streamlined. When getting started on your yoga practice, begin with the simplest version of the posture. Add more heat when you are ready.

In my classes, I begin with breathing for energy. There is nothing more basic than that. When raising your arms, keep going until your hands meet over your head and breathe. I then move to the neck and shoulders and down to the spine. Twists are good for the spine.

Do what you can. Do what you want. And practice.

> **"I'm really quite simple. I plant flowers and watch them grow... I stay at home and watch the river flow." – George Harrison**

Chapter 4

BODY PARTS

May the Force Be with You

In yoga, the force is your life force. When everything in life is going well, your life force is cursing through your body out into the world. You feel like you can handle anything. On bad days, you don't feel like you have any energy. You feel down and dull, too pooped to get out of bed, let alone get through the day. Still, your life force is there. It just needs to be sprung.

Your life force is stored in seven primary energy centers or chakras that are located along your spine up to the crown of your head. Each controls different physical and emotional functions. For example, the one behind your navel aids digestion and the one behind your heart controls your cardiovascular system and drives your compassion.

Certain postures, when practiced regularly, release the energy stored in your chakras. Breathing exercises help, too. For a quick fix, tap your thighs and feel the energy.

"You are responsible for the energy that you create for yourself, and you're responsible for the energy that you bring to others." – Oprah Winfrey

Head, Shoulders, Knees and Toes

The children's song "Head, Shoulders, Knees and Toes" is a good example of flow. While touching the part of the body referenced by the lyrics, there is movement. There is learning. And it is fun!

Have-A-Seat Yoga™ is fun, too. Rather than dictated by song, you focus on any part of the body that needs work or you let an instructor guide you if you are in a class. You might start at the top of your head and go to the bottom of your feet. The areas that need healing might be known to anyone you meet or invisible, known only to yourself.

With yoga we flow from one posture to the next, as we tone and strengthen our body. We learn to look inside ourselves, as we make room in our minds for peace. And, we laugh at ourselves when we realize we are holding our breath. You never want to hold your breath.

"Just play. Have fun. Enjoy the game." – Michael Jordan

All Fall Down

The nursey rhyme "Ring-a-round the Rosie," concludes with the line, "We all fall down," which is the cue for children to fall down laughing. For seniors, falling down is never something about which to laugh. Statistics published by the Centers for Disease Control (CDC) are scary and show that a fall often ends with a trip to the emergency room, a broken bone or two, lengthy rehabilitation, and a loss of independence.

Balance helps prevent falls, and Have-A-Seat Yoga™ helps improve your balance, both mentally and physically. Mentally, you learn to focus on the task at hand, even if the task is as simple as putting one foot in front of the other. Physically, you engage your abdominal muscles to strengthen your core, making many chores, whether you are in a chair or not, easier and safer. There are many postures and variations of postures to achieve a more balanced life.

"Life is like riding a bicycle. To keep your balance, you must keep moving." – Albert Einstein

Oh, My Aching Back

Do you suffer from back aches? Pain in the back slows you down and makes you feel old. Who needs it, but what can you do about it?

What about flabby arms, a thickening middle, or swollen ankles? And, you are probably wondering, where did those wrinkles come from?

As we get older, there's always something that bothers us about ourselves. Some of our problems arise from vanity. Others are a symptom of an underlying medical problem. You know which is which. If the later, see a doctor. If the former, practice Have-A-Seat Yoga™. You will boost your confidence. You might even lose some weight.

To repeat a well-known phrase: old age ain't for sissies. But we can make it easier on ourselves.

The Sanskrit word "dukkha" means pain or suffering. It incorporates the Buddhist concept that life is mundane and, therefore, unsatisfactory.

The Eyes Have It

While your mother might have told you to stop rolling your eyes when she was talking to you, eye rolling is a simple exercise to give your eyes a needed break. If you want to try it, sit straight in your chair and gaze up towards the ceiling without moving your head. Move your eyes to the right and back. Repeat three times and then close your eyes and relax. When you are ready, do it again by rolling your eyes to the left.

If your eyes are still tired, try palming by which you cover your eyes with your palms after you have warmed them by rubbing them together. This reduces visual stimulation and creates a blanket of darkness. Hold the position for a few seconds to up to five minutes.

These drills, as well as others, not only reduce eye strain, they also have other benefits: they direct your focus inward, bringing about a sense of well-being.

**"Behind every great man is
a woman rolling her eyes."
– Jim Carrey**

Make Like a Fish

Do you have a double chin? Many older people do. The collagen we lose as we age means our skin is not as smooth or as firm as it once was. You can't hide it, but you can fight it. Again, Have-A-Seat Yoga™ shows you the way.

Sitting in a chair, you can tone your neck muscles by tilting your head backwards and stroking your neck in a downwards motion. Then tilt you head forwards so that your chin touches your chest. Repeat.

Here's another exercise to give your jaw and neck a good stretch. Push your lower jaw out, and feel the tension. Hold for ten to fifteen seconds.

Or do the fish. It's not a dance; it's a facial posture which can be accomplished by sucking in your lips and checks until you start resembling a member of the aquatic species. Turn right, left, and up. Hold the pose and then repeat.

Of course, you can't undo the effects of a lifetime overnight, but you will see improvement over time.

"Life is like an ice-cream cone, you have to lick it one day at a time." – Charles M. Schulz

Pain in the Neck

There are many moves you can make in Have-A-Seat Yoga™ to rid you of the stress that has built up through the day in your neck, shoulders, and upper back.

As with yoga poses for the eyes, sit straight in your chair with your shoulders relaxed. First draw your chin towards your chest and then gently, always be gentle, roll your right ear toward your right shoulder. Then stretch by placing the fingertips of your left hand on your left shoulder and the fingertips of your right hand above your left ear. Count your breaths up to five and then switch sides. You are almost done, but you also want to roll your head from side to side for another five breaths.

You probably feel better already.

"The neck starts to go at 43, and that's that." – Nora Ephron

Bad Hair Day?

Hair was glorified in the musical *Hair*, first on and off Broadway and then in the movie. Women spend countless hours and money on their hair. We wash it. We style it. We cut it. We color it. If it is straight, we curl it. If it is curly, we straighten it. We pull it back or put it up. More and more men are doing the same.

If our hair looks good, we feel good, and our appearance is part of our well-being, as much as eating the right foods and getting enough sleep. We polish our nails, apply makeup, and carefully plan our wardrobe. Have-A-Seat Yoga™ gives us another leg up, as it makes us feel as if we can take on the world, no matter how we look.

> **"Anyone can be confident with a full head of hair. But a confident bald man–there's your diamond in the rough." – Larry David**

Prepare for Battle

In *Mad Max 2* (1981), Mel Gibson reprised his role as the title character to save a group of settlers from a gang of roving thugs. An embittered drifter who regained his humanity by doing good, he was known as "The Road Warrior."

The term "road warrior" today often refers to someone who travels extensively, usually for business. "Eco warrior" denotes an activist whose deeds are aimed at protecting the environment. In yoga, a warrior battles ignorance, especially from within.

The Warrior Pose, of which there are three variations and more options for the arms, has many benefits. It stretches the chest and lungs. It strengthens the shoulders, as well as the back muscles. While the pose is usually practiced while standing to build up leg muscles and stretch the thighs, calves, and ankles, these advantages can also be achieved when half-seated or when practicing Have-A-Seat Yoga™.

Traditionally, the "Warrior Pose" is called "Virabhadra's Pose." Virabhadra was a great warrior in Hindu mythology. The name comes from the Sanskrit word " vira" meaning "hero" and "bhadra" meaning "friend."

From the Ground Up

How often do you think about your feet? Unless you are trying on a new pair of shoes or cutting your toenails, the answer is probably not very often. Yet, our feet are so important. As the song says, "The foot bone connected to the leg bone," and so on. If you have foot problems, you suffer all over.

To give your feet a good workout, roll a tennis ball under each one for a few minutes. Pay attention to your toes, the ball of the foot, the arch, and the heel.

If you have taken off your shoes and socks, place a towel under your feet, scrunch your toes, and grab parts of the towel, slowly pulling it toward you.

If you prefer not to be barefoot, push down on your toes in your shoes and lift your heels off the ground. You will feel the stretch.

To strengthen your ankles, so important to mobility, move your feet, first one and then the other, in a circle with your legs extended. Do this ten to twenty times.

A good foot massage is one of life's little pleasures, and taking care of your feet during your practice or at any time is always time well spent.

> "I'm not into working out. My philosophy is no pain, no pain."
> – George Carlin

Chapter 5

PSYCH OUT

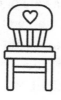

No Worries

Alfred E. Neuman, the boy mascot of *Mad* magazine, cheerfully proclaimed for decades, "What, me worry?" While this attitude appealed to generations of young people, no one can truthfully say that they don't have anything that bothers them, especially as they age.

For our mental health, we need peace and harmony, joy and humor, not simply satire and parody. We also need meaning in our lives. This comes from being aware of our needs, rising to challenges, and laughing at our mistakes.

Yoga won't make your troubles go away. However, when practiced regularly, either on the mat or in a chair, it will help you focus, so that you find a way to improve your situation.

It's not enough just to think about well-being, you have to work to be the best you can be, both mentally and physically, regardless of your circumstances.

What are you worried about? And what have you done about it?

"The reason why worry kills more people than work is that more people worry than work."
– Robert Frost

Follow the Bouncing Ball

Have you ever bounced back from a traumatic event in your life, one which you had thought had taken you to the point of no return? That's resilience, the ability to recover quickly from troubles. It is an important part of growth and change. Rather than seeing yourself as a victim, letting stress overwhelm you so can't cope or move ahead, you pick up the ball and run with it.

Resilience is not an inborn or genetic personality trait. It's a coping mechanism that can be developed over time. Having an upbeat outlook fosters resilience. So, too, does being optimistic, as well as controlling your emotions.

Have-A-Seat Yoga™ helps in all these areas. It nurtures a positive attitude toward yourself, so that you take care of yourself, even when bad things happen.

> **"I can be changed by what happens to me. But I refuse to be reduced by it."**
> **– Maya Angelou**

Game Changer

Game changers in sports are exciting. We cheer when a team intercepts the ball or a batter hits a tie-breaking home run. They happen when we least expect them, and we hold our breath as they play out, enjoying the thrill of the game.

In life, change is a constant, which we find disturbing and disruptive. As often as it happens, we are not prepared for it, and we resist it. Practicing Vinyasa yoga, on which Have-A-Seat Yoga™ is based, helps us get ready for a new normal that change has brought, whatever that new normal might be.

In yoga, we flow from one posture to the next and become stronger in body and spirit. We gain experience addressing change, and this experience has a positive impact on our lives. It's a game changer.

> **"If we don't change, we don't grow. If we don't grow, we aren't really living."**
> **– Gail Sheehy**

Keep Calm and Carry On

Is life getting you down? Do you find that you can't do everything you used to do or do it as well? If that's the case, think like the British: keep calm and carry on.

This expression appears on coffee mugs, t-shirts, refrigerator magnets, and other knick-knacks. Although it is sometimes attributed to Winston Churchill, which may or may not be true, it first appeared on a British government poster in 1939 to prepare the populace for World War II. Suggestive of that "stiff upper lip" for which our friends across the pond are known, it's as useful today as it ever was.

With Have-A-Seat Yoga™ , you can learn to address your troubles by developing a good attitude. In doing so, you will walk taller and feel better.

> **"Calm mind brings inner strength and self-confidence, so that's very important for good health." – Dalai Lama**

We Can Do It!

Americans had their own slogan to boost morale during World War II. The poster with the female factory worker known as "Rosie the Riveter," who, flexing her well-developed arm, looked determined and unwavering, reminds us that we have the resilience and strength to accomplish what we set out to do. "We can do it!" Rosie declares. Or, as the shoe company Nike tells us, "Just Do It." Have a seat and do it!

> **"Optimism is the faith that leads to achievement. Nothing can be done without hope and confidence." – Helen Keller**

I Want to Thank...

As part of the Academy Awards Ceremony, not that many of us watch anymore, the acceptance speeches almost always include a list of those people who enabled the winners, be they actors or those behind the scenes, to go on stage to receive their Oscar. It's a tradition.

While these folks may or may not be sincere when they express their appreciation for the help they received along the way, true gratitude has a positive impact on our well-being. It centers on all the good things in life and lifts our spirit. It might be for something as fleeting as a child's kiss on the cheek or as long-lasting as a good marriage.

Incorporate gratitude into your yoga practice with every breath you take. Every day write down something for which you are thankful or someone who made your day better. At night review your list. You will sleep better.

The Sanskrit word "kritajna" means gratitude. It connotes being fully present, acknowledging a moment in time.

Counting Sheep

You gain many benefits when you include meditation in your practice.

You don't stop thinking during meditation. By organizing your thoughts, so they stop bumping into each other, you make space in your mind to value new experiences.

By centering your mind, you generate emotional and mental stability, alleviating symptoms of depression and anxiety.

By focusing your thoughts, you release creative energy.

By freeing your mind, you achieve a brief respite from your problems.

By looking inward, you gain greater awareness of yourself, as well as those around you. You appreciate your life and everyone in it.

Regular meditation brings balance and growth. You develop a general sense of well-being, so you fall asleep easier when you go to bed and stay asleep throughout the night. No more counting sheep.

"I close my eyes in order to see."
– Paul Gauguin

Let Me Count the Ways

There are different ways to meditate.

If you are sitting on a mat, you can fold your legs in a lotus position or stretch them out in front of you. If you are in a chair, you can drop your arms to the side or fold them in your lap. Regardless of your position, you want to be comfortable so that you can relax, but not so comfortable that you fall asleep.

You also need to decide what to do with your hands. Gestures, called "mudras," channel energy through your body. For example, the gesture called "chin," which looks like the okay symbol, is created by putting the index finger under the tip of the thumb and extending the remaining three fingers. There are others.

Finally, you want to dispel your thoughts, be they good or bad. Saying a mantra, such as "om" or chanting a theme of your own helps concentration. You might want to focus on a chakra or gaze at a lit candle. Some people prefer to meditate when moving about. Mindful walking, whereby you are aware of every step you take and conscious of how it feels, is another way of clearing your mind so that you can look within.

The Sanskrit word "padmassana" refers to the lotus position, whereby one crosses their legs and places their feet on their opposing thighs.

Singing the Blues

Cats are so entertaining we watch hours of cat videos on the Internet. Their climbing and curiosity mesmerize and delight us.

Cats, too, are great company. Cats, like dogs, lower stress and help us cope. If you need a cuddle, they're there for you. Well, maybe that's not always so. They might be chasing a ball of yarn or planning a stupid pet trick.

If you're feeling blue, pet a cat. This works if you're a cat person. If you're not, play some jazz or practice Have-A-Seat Yoga™.

> **"For me, singing sad songs often has a way of healing a situation. It gets the hurt out in the open into the light, out of the darkness." – Reba McEntire**

Color Your World

In recent years, people have discovered the joy of coloring, and adult coloring books have become a craze, one that brings creativity and calm to its devotees.

Color impacts our emotions and behavior. In yoga, a color is associated with each of the seven primary chakras or energy centers that run along the spine. We can choose how we want to feel and what we want to accomplish by breathing a color and imagining it saturating our body.

To feel stable and connected, breath red.

To unleash originality and sexuality, breath orange.

To develop your sense of self, breath yellow. Yellow is associated with power and action.

If you are feeling poorly, breath green, and you will help heal yourself. You will also feel more compassion, as well as joy.

If you want to improve your communications by expressing yourself truthfully, think of the sky and breath blue.

To feel calm and improve your intuition, breath indigo, another color of the rainbow.

Violet, the color associated with the seventh chakra at the top of your head, represents spiritual illumination. Breathing violet will help you achieve perspective, if not enlightenment.

> **"Gardening is how I relax. It's another form of creating and playing with colors." – Oscar de la Renta**

Chapter 6

THE SOCIAL NETWORK

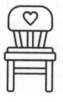

The French Connection

Do you salivate when you think of a chocolate-filled croissant? Does your heart race when you know you're running late? Do you relax as soon as you immerse yourself in a hot bubble bath? The mind and body connection exists.

One effects the other. Your aches and pain influence your thinking. If you are stressed, you are more likely to make mistakes.

Conversely, your thinking impacts your behavior. If you are unsure of yourself, you often put off making a decision. If you feel confident, nothing will get in the way of your success.

Yoga is a mental and physical practice. When we flow from one posture to another, we get a good workout. We meditate to clear our minds and give us control over our postures. We go deep inside ourselves to reach out to the world. Conscious breathing ties it all together, and we make connections.

"Man consists of two parts,
his mind and his body, only
the body has more fun."
— Woody Allen

Keep in Touch

When we want to know what is happening outside of our circle of friends, we go on the Internet, turn on the television, or pick up a newspaper. Yes, an old-fashioned newspaper, one you can hold in your hands. The news gives us something to talk about. It might be something as silly as celebrity gossip or as consuming as a sports score. More importantly, it keeps us informed about the events that impact our lives.

We also need to be connected on a personal level. This means feeling a sense of belonging and being accepted for who we are. We seek consistency, support, trust, and love, especially when the news isn't good or life isn't going our way.

If you are looking to make connections, but you are not ready to give as well as receive, to admit your mistakes or ask for advice, practice Have-A-Seat Yoga™ with a partner or simply join hands with the person sitting next to you.

"Wherever I am, it's a really good feeling to have that connection to people. I love to go out to talk to people and be with folks. I don't shy away from it." – Danny DeVito

R–E–S–P– E–C–T

Relationships are built on respect. Through Have-A-Seat Yoga™ , we learn respect. We find that we are the same, despite our differences. We learn that no one is perfect, and we develop compassion. We make connections, so no one is left behind. We create energy, and we send it out into the world. So, first of all, respect yourself.

At school, respect your teacher, although you won't necessarily get better grades.

At work, respect your boss, your colleagues, your subordinates, although it won't guarantee a promotion or a raise.

At home, respect your spouse, your parents, your children, your friends. It will improve your quality of life.

Wherever you are, respect everyone around you and everyone who came before you. It's your past and present. It might also be your future.

Respect your community, the environment, the planet. It's your world, and you can make it a better place.

"I'm not concerned with
your liking or disliking me...
All I ask is that you respect
me as a human being."
– Jackie Robinson

Lost in Translation

Talk a little. Talk a lot. One-on-one communication is a two-way street, no matter how much is said or left unsaid. One person imparts information, and the second person responds. Good communication is based on active giving and taking. It's how we connect.

Here's an exercise you can do with a partner or a friend to see how well you communicate. Sit side by side, not looking at each other. One person begins by describing their week, and then the other plays back what they "heard." If you are the speaker, ask yourself: "Is that what I was trying to say? Is that what I was feeling?" Maybe. Maybe not.

Listening is particularly important. If you are the receiver, how do you know that you heard what you were supposed to hear?

Was there a connection? Maybe. Maybe not. Whether speaking or responding, you need to think before you act.

Maybe you want to try again.

"The single biggest problem
in communication is the
illusion that it has taken place."
– George Bernard Shaw

Let's Talk Turkey

The world turns. Thursday is the new Friday. Orange is the new black. Fifty is the new forty. Do you even know what these expressions mean?

"On" and "off" used to apply to the light switch, as in: "Please turn on the lights." Of course, people who lived by candlelight at night, think Abraham Lincoln, wouldn't have a clue what you were talking about. Similarly, people who have never been on the Internet don't know the difference between online and offline.

To stay in touch with what's happening outside, go to your children and grandchildren. The language they use speaks volumes.

With age comes wisdom based on experience. We have learned lessons that we want to share, but sometimes it is best to listen. Teach your children well. And they will teach you.

**"Slang is a language that rolls up
its sleeves, spits on its hands and
goes to work." – Carl Sandburg**

The Ties that Bind

As long as we have watched television, we have laughed and cried with the Ricardos, the Cleavers, the Nelsons, the Petries, the Bradys, the Bunkers, the Jeffersons, the Keatons, the Huxtables, the Bundys, and the Bluths. We lamented the cancellation of *Roseanne*, even if we felt it was rightly deserved, but the family might survive in a show called "The Conners." The family always survives.

Sometimes we feel that our own family is fodder for a sitcom, if not an hour-long drama that plays out day after day, week after week. Still, the family, flawed or not, is considered the basic unit of civilization. We return to our family after a demanding day at work, a losing fight on the playground, or exchanging harsh words with a friend. Families offer support and comfort. Families represent our roots, helping us be grounded and connected.

So, make peace with your siblings. Visit with your children. Enjoy your grandchildren. Take care of your parents. Find your way home.

"The oldest form of theater is the dinner table. It's got five or six people, new show every night, same players. Good ensemble; the people have worked together a lot."
– Michael J. Fox

Linking up

Doing research on one's background has become very popular. You can explore your genealogy and create your family tree. You can purchase a DNA kit online or over the phone. Interest in the past is a very good thing. Now, take it a step further, and impart your family stories to your children and grandchildren.

Research conducted at Emory University shows that "Family stories provide a sense of identity through time, and help children understand who they are in the world." They know they belong to something bigger than themselves. The more children know about their background, the better their emotional health, the more resilient they are coping with stress.

If you are not sure where to begin, try writing down what you remember. Were your grandparents present in your life when you were growing up? What do you know about their lives? Where did they come from? How did they meet? Now, what about your parents? What about you?

Similar to taking a yoga class, sharing one's stories is a powerful means of connection.

"If you don't know your family's history, then you don't know anything. You are like a leaf that doesn't know it is part of a tree." – Michael Crichton

Birds of a Feather

Do you have a friend that is always complaining? On one hand, you might empathize with your friend and want to keep your friend company in his or her misery. On the other hand, he or she is probably bringing you down.

I'm sure you are a good friend. However, a negative friendship can impair one's mental health, while a positive friendship, one based on kindness and honesty, brings happiness and good feelings.

Have-A-Seat Yoga™ is a way to find a new path, one that helps you find solutions and solve problems, rather than compounding bad situations. It is also a way to meet people with whom you share a deeper bond.

It's never too late to make new friends. It takes effort and time, but it's worth it.

> **"A friend is a gift you give yourself." – Robert Louis Stevenson**

Best Friend Forever

The acronym "BFF" has been around longer than you think. In a 1997 episode of "Friends," Phoebe explained it to her friends. It made an appearance as a noun in *The New Oxford Dictionary* in 2010, but there's no reason to look it up. We all know what it means.

If we have a falling out with our best friend, or any friend, it's traumatic. Still, we survive. As we grow older, we realize that it is very unusual to keep our friends throughout our lives. There are reasons for this. We move away or move on to different activities or interests. We don't put in the time or effort, and we lose touch.

Still, friends are important to our well-being, possibly even better for us than family. Similar to Have-A-Seat Yoga™, they insulate us from fear of getting older and alleviate stress.

Like Waldo, your new best friends might be hiding in a crowd scene. It's up to you to find them.

"There are no strangers here; only friends you haven't yet met." – William Butler Yeats

Join Up

By "join up" I don't mean "enlist." You're probably too old anyway. I mean "connect."

We all need to connect with something, with someone. If we don't we'll be very lonely.

Social media, be it Facebook or Twitter or a new app, isn't a cure for loneliness, but it gives us a way to connect, to share accomplishments and photos, to reach out to old friends and make new ones.

Volunteering also gives us a way to connect – to young people, to old people, to anyone in trouble needing help, to people helping other people.

As important as feeling connected is as we age, volunteering does more than that. When we use our skills, we develop new skills. When we share our experiences, we gain new experiences. If we engage in physical labor, we improve our health.

Through Have-A-Seat Yoga™ we find the way. And we find the time to give back.

The Sanskrit word "dāna" means giving.

Chapter 7

DO BE DO BE DO

Do Sing Out

With a focus on etiquette and doing the right thing, Romper Room, a children's television show that ran from 1953 to 1994, promoted its message with the "Do Bee a Do Bee" theme song. "Do be a sidewalk player. Do be a car sitter. Do be a plate cleaner," the song counseled, as well as pointed out what you shouldn't be. There was also a dance with its own song. "Buzz. Buzz," make like a bee. Everyone was encouraged to join in.

There are so many good things that you can do to enhance your practice and improve your well-being. Some suggestions follow. Pick and choose, or do your own thing.

"To do is to be."
– Jean-Paul Sartre

Do Open Up

When you are open to new people, new ideas, and new experiences, good things will come your way.

Have an open-ended conversation whereby no one has an agenda, hidden or otherwise, and make a new friend.

Spend an open-ended day with nothing on your schedule. Without the stress of having to be some place at a given time, you'll enjoy yourself.

Take to the open road, even if it's only in your mind, and see where it leads.

Open a door to discover what's on the other side.

Seek out wide open spaces where you have room to grow and dream.

Open your eyes. Appreciate the beauty around you.

Open your heart with gentle twists. If you can, do a simple backbend. Inhale slowly and smoothly. Let in love.

If you are deciding whether Have-A-Seat Yoga™ is for you, keep an open mind.

"A mind is like a parachute. It doesn't work if it is not open."
— Frank Zappa

Do Clean Up

Clean off your plate. Clean out your closet. Clean off your desk. Clean up your act. Cleanliness is next to godliness, and you've been cleaning up, sometimes after yourself and often after others, your whole life. Now, as you continue to do so, clean your mind.

I'm not suggesting that you have a dirty mind, but, in all likelihood, it is messy. It contains all the things on your to-do list, the many items in your closet that you've been meaning to give away, the last unpleasant conversation you had with someone close to you or an argument you had with your neighbor. You know you were right or that's what you keep telling yourself. Some of the clutter is good. Use it. Release the bad. Let it go.

"When I'm not in my right mind, my left mind gets pretty crowded." – Steven Wright

Do Space Out

Make space for your practice. While yoga can be practiced anywhere, even outdoors, you'll want to have a special place for when you meditate at home.

This special place can be a room or a corner of a room. It should be free from distractions and clutter. The light should be abundant, and outside noise should be minimal. There should be space for your accessories, including a chair and a pillow, maybe a blanket. Add a few personal items, such as candles, seashells, chimes, or an easy-to-care plant.

Aromatherapy can help you relax when you meditate. The oils, such as lavender, smell good, too. Keep some nearby, and take a deep breath or rub some on your wrists before you cool down.

Your space should make you happy to be there.

"We must still think of ourselves
as pioneers to understand
the importance of space."
– Buzz Aldrin

Do Bring It On

Good morning, sunshine. It's a new day. If you have been practicing Have-A-Seat Yoga™, you are ready for just about anything. You slept well. Your hip doesn't hurt. You feel confident.

Once you are awake, you might want to begin your activities with a sun salutation, a series of postures to warm your body and get you moving. It can be a warm-up to your routine or it can be your entire routine. It can be done slowly which is calming or quickly which is stimulating. Focus for a few minutes on the sun, and express your gratitude for the light which embraces you. Then rest and go, prepared for whatever comes your way.

The Sanskrit term "Surya Namaskar" refers to the series of postures which comprise the Sun Salutation.

Do Take Off

If you've never practiced yoga, think of Have-A-Seat Yoga™ as a journey. As you get ready, you have lots of questions, as you would for any trip you are planning. Some of these might be:

Where do I want to go?

Should I travel by myself or go with a partner?

When will I leave?

How long will I be away?

What should I take with me?

The answers are up to you. You might want to go to the end of the line and plan on leaving right away. Simply remember to travel light, and be sure to bring your curiosity and enthusiasm.

> **"What draws me in is that a trip is a leap in the dark. It's like a metaphor for life. You set off from home, and in the classic travel book, you go to an unknown place. You discover a different world, and you discover yourself." — Paul Theroux**

Do Double Down

To double your blackjack winnings, split pairs, except for aces and eights, or take one card when your first two cards total ten or eleven. The odds are in your favor.

To double your pleasure, have a stick of Doublemint gum.

To double your trouble, date twins.

To see double, have one too many cocktails. Beware of a hangover.

To impress your friends, accept a double dare.

To double your fun, practice Have-A-Seat Yoga™ with a friend. It's always better to share.

"Yabba dabba do."
– Fred Flintstone

Do Jump In

The water's fine, but you won't know this if you are sitting at the edge of the pool, simply admiring the view. Take off your shoes. Wiggle your toes. Now, put them in the water. Ahhhhh.

If you have taken the plunge and attended your first Have-A-Seat Yoga™ session good for you! Now go all in.

> **"Only when the tide goes out do you discover who's been swimming naked."**
> **– Warren Buffett**

Do Break Out

Your yoga practice need never be boring.

You can try new postures, make modifications, and change the sequence. You can also vary your practice by time of day. In the morning, spend your routine by warming your muscles and joints. In the evening, work on your balance and unwind from the problems you encountered during the day.

The seasons, too, offer a reason to change what you do. In the winter, when it is cold and dark, sun salutations can cheer you up and generate energy. In warm, sunny environments, twists and forward bends help you stay cool, calm, and collected, when you might otherwise be agitated and out of sorts.

> **"Only I can change my life.**
> **No one can do it for me."**
> **– Carol Burnett**

Do Make Up

"Love means never having to say you're sorry." But what does love have to do with it? Sometimes when things go wrong, intentionally or accidentally, a simple apology resolves the situation. Not everyone will hear your apology nor accept it, but it begins a conversation. It helps if you are sincere.

It takes courage to say "I'm sorry." So gather your courage and admit your mistakes. Taking responsibility feels good.

Conversely, it is up to you to accept an apology. It's a two-way street.

Now, kiss and make up.

> **"If you're going to do something tonight that you'll be sorry for tomorrow morning, sleep late."**
> — Henny Youngman

Chapter 8

DON'T STOP

Don't Stop Practicing

In life, as well as yoga, practice makes perfect. Although you may never reach your goals, the effort is worth it. Here are some suggestions on what you might want to avoid on your path to well-being.

At the top of the list is to do no harm – to yourself or others. It's the first of the eight limbs of yoga, as put forth in the *Yoga Sutras*, compiled by the Hindu mystic Patanjali.

If you feel pain or discomfort when you are holding a pose, relax. Maybe, move on to the next pose in your sequence. If you are angry with someone, let go of your thoughts. Turn your negative thoughts into something positive. Be a friend.

"Ahimsa", derived from Sanskrit, means non-violence.

Don't Be Cruel

Elvis Presley recorded "Don't Be Cruel" in 1956. He performed the song during his three appearances on *The Ed Sullivan Show*.

The song has messages for today. Even its title encourages kindness and consideration, so much a part of Have-A-Seat Yoga™.

It laments loneliness: "Well, you know I can be found, sitting all alone."

It promotes communication: "If you can't come around, at least, please telephone."

It offers an apology: "If I made you mad, for something I might have said…"

It encourages commitment: "Let's walk to the preacher. Let's say, hey, I do."

"Hound Dog" was on the flip side. "Don't Be Cruel" overtook "Hound Dog," itself a best-selling single, to rise to number one on all three music charts: pop, country, and R and B. There's another message here: don't be a hound dog crying all the time."

"No act of kindness, no matter how small, is ever wasted." – Aesop

Don't Be a Party Pooper

If someone smiles at you, smile back.

If someone asks you to dance, dance.

If someone is going for a ride, go along and spring for gas.

If someone invites you to lunch, go to lunch.

If someone offers you a piece of cake, help yourself.

If someone wants to know your opinion, tell them what you think.

If someone tells a joke, clap your hands and laugh out loud. If you don't get it, that's something else.

If someone invites you to a party, ask what you can bring and put on your party clothes. You don't have to be the life of the party, but you don't have to be a wallflower either.

> **"The good life is a process, not a state of being. It is a direction not a destination."**
> **– Carl Rogers**

Don't Be a Stranger

There are many ways to say "goodbye." "Ta ta" is informal and attributed to the British during World War II. TTFN, meaning "goodbye for now," is often used when texting. If you use the French phrase "au revoir" you are saying, "until we meet again."

If a colleague is changing jobs, a fellow practitioner takes another class, or a neighbor moves across town, it is difficult to say "goodbye." "Don't be a stranger" is a way to say, "Stay in touch."

You need to do the same. At some point, everyone moves on. This doesn't mean you lose a friend, not if you reach out. And if you are open, you will make a new one.

> **"Make new friends, but keep the old. One is silver, and the other gold." – Girl Scouts of the USA**

Don't Be Late

If you are taking a class, think of all you miss if you are just a few minutes late, such as the quiet time and the warm up.

Showing up late is simply rude. It indicates a complete disregard for others, and it is the antithesis of yoga. You disturb your fellow practitioners, as they have to move their mats or chairs to make room for you. You interrupt the sequence that your teacher has set into motion. You disrupt the calmness and serenity that has been generated. The energy just seeps out of the room.

If you are late, don't make excuses. No one wants to hear them.

> **"Manners are a sensitive awareness of the feelings of others. If you have that awareness, you have good manners, no matter what fork you use." – Emily Post**

Don't Be a Stiff

Why would you ever stop stretching? It feels so good, and it is good for you, too.

Actors stretch when they take on a role. Musicians stretch when they compose a song. Chefs stretch when they try a recipe or add a new ingredient. And they grow.

Stretching relieves tension. Stretching keeps your muscles limber and loose. It improves flexibility and increases circulation. By maintaining a range of motion you have better coordination. You stand straighter, too, minimizing your aches and pains.

Stretch your shoulders, neck, and lower back. Don't forget your calves, hamstrings, and hips, so important for mobility.

Have-A-Seat Yoga™ may or may not help you stretch your budget, but it can certainly help you stretch your mind and tone your body.

> **"Stretching was a major part of my preparation."**
> **– Edwin Moses**

Don't Stop Laughing

Children are easily amused. A funny face or a knock-knock joke brings peals of laughter to the playground. The class clown is often one of the popular kids, known for his or her quips and tricks, rather than scholastics. Unfortunately, as we get older, we feel it is more appropriate to keep a straight face, and we become more serious. This is too bad.

Laughter is a wonderful thing. It has physical, mental, and social benefits. It relaxes our muscles, relieves stress, and brings us closer to others.

Laughter might not replace yoga practice or going to the gym, but it is good for your health.

If there's nothing else to laugh about, laugh at yourself – or make up a knock-knock joke.

"A day without laughter is a day wasted." – Charlie Chaplin

Don't Watch the Clock

Time never stands still. If we are having fun, we wonder where the time went. As we get older, time seems to fly by. We ask ourselves: What happened to yesterday? Last week? Last month? Last year? What about the last decade? Looking back, it feels as if nothing happened.

One theory for this phenomena is that as adults we settle into a routine and our day-to-day experiences blur together. A suggested antidote is to create new memories, to make new friends, to learn something new, to try something unusual.

You can't stop time, but you can take advantage of it.

> 'The time is always right to do what is right.' – Martin Luther King, Jr.

Don't Be Afraid

What are you afraid of?

Are you afraid of looking in the mirror? If you had a late night, you probably want to avoid a mirror.

Are you afraid of getting older? Well, we all get older. There's little you can do about it.

Do you avoid trying something new? If you don't try it, you won't know that you like it.

When you start Have-A-Seat Yoga™, you can't lose. Even if you feel foolish when wiggling your toes or waving your arms, it's a win-win situation. You will feel better, and you add your energy to that of fellow practitioners.

Don't cower in the closet. instead, confront your fears. It's a good way of banishing them.

> **"Never let the fear of striking out keep you from playing the game." – Babe Ruth**

Don't Hold Your Breath

Nothing good ever comes when you hold your breath. In fact, your breath is the basis of your yoga practice. It unites the body, mind, and spirit. In Have-A-Seat Yoga™, you learn to control your breath and breathe consciously.

Breathing consciously enhances awareness, so you connect with your feelings while you meditate.

Breathing consciously advances relaxation, giving you time to recharge. We all need a break.

Breathing consciously produces balance, so you are both energized and calm, creative and grounded. When you breathe slower or faster, you change your state of mind.

Breathing consciously creates energy, and the energy moves through your body freely. You feel alive in the moment.

> **"I took a deep breath and
> listened to the old bray of
> my heart. I am. I am. I am."**
> **– Sylvia Plath**

Chapter 9

KEEP IT GOING

Stay Positive

You never want to give up – on yourself, your family, or your friends. We all hit road-blocks. Some are small while others seem monumental. Even when it is dark, remember the Johnny Mercer and Harold Arlen song: "Accentuate the positive, eliminate the negative."

There are numerous ways, one of which is yoga, to get to the right place where there is hope.

Yoga helps you put your problems into perspective. With meditation, you can find solutions to your problems. As you become stronger, both mentally and physically, you have the strength to address your problems.

If you have started Have-A-Seat Yoga™, here are suggestions to take the lessons you learned out of the chair and into your life, and keep it going.

"Failure happens all the time. It happens every day in practice. What makes you better is how you react to it." — Mia Hamm

Have Patience

Change doesn't come all at once.

It is difficult to change yourself. Anyone who has gone on a diet knows that. And those back aches don't disappear overnight.

It is difficult to change attitudes. The argument you had with your daughter lingers in your mind far longer than it should. Were you wrong? Was she wrong? Ask yourself what difference does it make.

If you are finding it difficult to practice, maybe you need to take a break. Everyone needs a break, even if they are doing something they love. Or, better yet, maybe you just need to change your routine.

With the right attitude and practice, good things will happen.

Every day is a new day. Keep smiling.

**"The more I practice the luckier
I get." – Arnold Palmer**

Get in the Mood

If you are trying to decide whether to practice, music can put you in the mood. After all, sound is a vibration, similar to reciting a mantra, and it impacts our emotions and affects our environment.

Not all types of music are suited for yoga or inspire meditation. Many people enjoy classical Indian music, which has regional variations, when they are practicing. Ravi Shankar popularized the sound of the sitar, a stringed instrument, and many rock bands incorporated it into hit songs. The tabla, a percussion instrument consisting of two drums, is often used to keep the beat.

More familiar classical music can be calming. Ambient music, with sounds of nature, such as waves breaking, birds singing, or rain falling, creates a soothing background.

Alternatively, there is always silence.

"Music does a lot of things for a lot of people. It's transporting, for sure. It can take you right back, years back, to the very moment certain things happened in your life. It's uplifting, it's encouraging, it's strengthening."
– Aretha Franklin

Join the Party

International Yoga Day, declared by the United Nations in 2015, is June 21. At its inception in India, almost 36,000 practitioners, representing eighty-four nations, performed twenty-one postures for thirty-five minutes on Rajpath, a grassy boulevard in New Delhi. Millions around the world observed the event, doing their own thing.

Several years later, the celebration has grown, and more and more people, be they young or old, fat or thin, male or female, from different backgrounds join together to mark the day. In Washington DC, they gather on Capitol Hill. In New York City, the Statue of Liberty provides an inspiring backdrop. It's a perfect time to go to a park, breathe fresh air, join other yogis, and learn what yoga is all about.

> **"One cannot have too large
> a party. A large party
> secures its own amusement."**
> **– Jane Austen**

Form a Circle

Circle games are played at birthday parties to involve all participants equally or used as icebreakers when adults get together.

The "Circle of Life' in Disney's *The Lion King* is sung as a tribute to the young lion Simba when he is introduced to the animals in the kingdom.

Creating a mandala, a complex and abstract design, brings us focus. In Buddhism, it is believed to lead to enlightenment.

Yoga circles are gaining in popularity as practitioners seek a sense of belonging.

Circles are universal and have meaning beyond their geometric form. They represent wholeness, unity, and harmony. They can be found in nature, but sometimes we have to fashion them for ourselves. Bring your family, friends, and even strangers into your circle.

The Sanskrit word "mandala" means circle.

Keep a Journal

Inspire yourself. Keep a journal of your Have-A-Seat Yoga™ sessions, and refer to it when you don't think you want to practice.

You don't need to spend a lot of time on this activity, unless your words are flowing. Bullet points work well, if you are in a hurry. You needn't worry about grammar or punctuation. This is for you.

Write about the practical aspects of the session. The topics you cover might include the day of the week and the time of day you practiced, how long you practiced, the poses you had trouble with, and the poses you undertook with ease. In other words, keep track of what and when.

In your journal, you can also explore your thoughts and feelings. Here you might note how you felt before, during, and after practice, or what your thoughts were during meditation. Many people also use their journals to write about the things for which they are grateful. You can do the same.

When you look back on how far you have come in your practice, you will be impressed, and you will want to keep going.

"Writing is an exploration. You start from nothing and learn as you go." – E. L. Doctorow

Read a Book

Reading is relaxing. It has other benefits, too. It expands your vocabulary and improves your memory. It is exercise for the mind.

Read any books that interest you. If you read non-fiction, whatever the subject, you will undoubtedly learn something new. If you enjoy fiction, be it the classics or the latest bestsellers, you will delve into the minds and emotions of others, becoming more empathetic.

If you want to be a writer, read.

If you want to go to new places but can no longer travel, read.

If you want to expand your yoga practice, read.

Motivate yourself to read by browsing in a library or an online bookstore or by joining a book club. Take a book with you when you have a cup of coffee. Sip and enjoy.

"With every book, you go back
to school. You become a student.
You become an investigative
reporter. You spend a little
time learning what it's like to
live in someone else's shoes."
– John Irving

Practice Mindfulness

We all lead busy lives. We cannot afford to be distracted. Many have found relief from stress from their many responsibilities by practicing mindfulness.

Mindfulness is more than the latest self-help fad. It's the art of being present. Practice mindfulness when you wake up and go about your usual routine, and you will enjoy the rest of your day. Whatever you are doing, whether it is taking a shower, eating breakfast, talking to a neighbor, notice everything around you – the smells, the tastes, the feelings you encounter.

You can train yourself to be mindful. It won't happen overnight, but you can do it in increments. When you find your mind wandering, gently bring it back to the task at hand, whether you are minding the store or sitting in traffic. If you are plugged into your cell phone, turn it off. Doing too many things at once is the antithesis of mindfulness.

Be mindful when you practice Have-A-Seat Yoga™. Do a forward bend and take pleasure in the stretch. You'll want to do it again and again.

> "The moment one gives close
> attention to anything, even
> a blade of grass, it becomes
> a mysterious, awesome,
> indescribably magnificent world
> in itself." – Henry Miller

Talk the Talk

Language is used to communicate. We speak, we listen, we read, and we write.

Language is part of culture. When we travel, we learn a second language, or some phrases and words, so that we feel more comfortable during our visit.

Have-A-Seat Yoga™ is also a journey, and learning Sanskrit, the language of yoga, takes you to another place so you better appreciate the philosophy of yoga, understand why you are practicing, and realize what you hope to accomplish.

The type of yoga you practice tells you something about your practice. For example, Hatha yoga is a style of yoga that emphasizes the postures. "Hatha" means force, although, generally the practice is relatively gentle. "Ha" means sun and "tha" means moon, and we learn to balance as we practice. Ashtanga means eight limbs or branches of yoga of which asana, the physical component, is merely one branch of the practice.

All asanas or postures also have Sanskrit names.

"I personally think we
developed language because
of our deep need to complain."
– Lily Tomlin

Live the Life

Maybe, you once dreamed of equipping your kitchen with stainless steel appliances, remodeling your bathroom with Italian fixtures, or revving the engine of your luxury automobile. Now you've downsized and taken up yoga. You wake up in the morning and look forward to your practice. You go to class and get in the flow. You practice breathing consciously. All told, you feel better about yourself.

Yoga, however, is more than exercise. To keep it going, you can make it a lifestyle. To help you on your journey, the Yoga Sutras, a guide for living the good life, prescribes eight aspects or limbs to follow. These include developing high moral standards and imposing self-discipline. You probably follow many of the principles laid out in this ancient text every day. After all, you are a good person. Still, learning more about yoga will be inspiring. It will certainly give you something to think about.

"Nonviolence is not a garment to put on and off at will. Its seat is in the heart, and it must be an inseparable part of our very being." – Mahatma Gandhi

Chapter 10

STUDIES SHOW

Help for the Common Cold

When you have a runny nose and feel achy and miserable, you probably have a cold. Experience tells you to drink plenty of fluids and rest. Mild to moderate exercise might help reduce your symptoms, although you might want to stay in bed.

When you have a cold, you are contagious. You certainly should not go to work and your yoga instructor will not be pleased to see you in class. Still, there are yoga postures you can do at home to make you feel better. A simple forward bend helps clear sinuses. A spinal twist rids organs of unwanted toxins. A resting pose energizes and relaxes.

While proof that yoga cures colds is lacking, there are many research studies that show that yoga is the antidote for what ails you, whether you have chronic back problems or pain from osteoarthritis. Some ailments which you might be experiencing and the way yoga lessens your pain are reviewed in the following sections.

"If you take a reasonable amount of vitamin C regularly, the incidence of the common cold goes down. If you get a cold and start immediately, as soon as you start sneezing and sniffling, the cold just doesn't get going." – Linus Pauling

Help for Back Pain

Do you have trouble moving around? Are you walking slower than you used to? Do you have pain in your lower back? Is it a dull ache or does a stabbing pain come on suddenly? As put forth in *NIH Research Matters*, studies have shown that yoga is a useful treatment for relieving discomfort, not only for middle-class adults, but among those from lower income backgrounds, as well.

In one study, test subjects were divided into three groups: one attended yoga sessions, one received physical therapy, and one received educational materials on self-care. All three groups experienced pain reduction, but those who practiced yoga or received physical therapy were significantly more likely to stop taking pain relievers after one year.

Put a twist to the spine to not only relieve tension in your back, but your neck, as well. Bend backwards, forwards, or move in a circle. Draw one knee to your chest and return it to the floor. Now do the same on the other. You will undo the problems brought on by sitting all day long.

"Find a place inside where there's joy, and the joy will burn out the pain."
– Joseph Campbell

Help for Osteoarthritis

A small study conducted at Florida Atlantic University and first published in the *Journal of the American Geriatrics Society* in December 2016 showed there is a positive association between practicing chair yoga and some of the debilitating effects of osteoarthritis in the lower extremities.

A test group of sixty-five persons participated in two forty-five-minute weekly sessions of chair yoga for eight weeks while a control group attended a health education program for the same duration. Measurements for pain, balance, walking speed, and fatigue taken at the beginning of the study were compared at the middle and end of the study showed reduction in the amount of pain and fatigue, as well as an improvement in gait.

But you have to keep it up. Any improvements were lost per measurements taken one and three months after classes had ended.

"I don't deserve this award,
but I have arthritis and I
don't deserve that either."
– Jack Benny

Help for Insomnia

Do you check the clock? Do you pull up the comforter? Do you turn on your side? Do you check the clock – again? You're having another sleepless night. Wil you ever catch up on your sleep?

The benefits of a good night's sleep are well known. Sleep gives us energy and aids our memory. Sleep has healing powers, and it puts us in a better mood. Unfortunately, our ability to get a good night's sleep decreases with age.

There are many tips for getting a good night's sleep. Don't drink coffee before bedtime. In fact, stay away from alcohol, too. It acts as a stimulant. Water only leads to more trips to the bathroom. Nor, should you eat late in the day. You don't want indigestion when you are trying to fall asleep. Create the right environment in your bedroom, one that is quiet and comfortable. Relax, and clear your mind. Although there are no definitive studies that demonstrate the impact of yoga on sleep, yoga, with its emphasis on breathing and meditation, helps.

"The best cure for insomnia is to get a lot of sleep." – W. C. Fields

Help for Fatigue

Do you often feel tired at some point during the day? Sometimes it is just a change in your routine. Maybe, you skipped breakfast or your usual exercise. Possibly, you haven't had enough water to drink or you suffer from iron deficiency. Perhaps, you didn't sleep well the night before or you are stressed and worried.

Chronic fatigue is an on-going problem for many. It might be a sign of a medical condition for which you need to see a doctor. There is both physical fatigue, whereby your muscles are sore, and mental fatigue, whereby you find it difficult to concentrate. Physical and mental fatigue are different, but they could be related.

Cancer survivors often experience fatigue, impacting their quality of life. As reported in the *Journal of Clinical Oncology*, a research study showed that those of the 410 study participants who received standard care plus yoga instruction twice a week for seventy-five minutes per session had significantly reduced fatigue and an improved quality of life when compared to a control group.

The yoga sessions focused on breathing exercises and consisted of gentle postures and meditation.

> **"I am just a little tired of the
> Stones and the Beatles, and
> I don't care if I ever hear
> 'Louie Louie' ever again."
> – Wolfman Jack**

Help for Headaches

Peppermint, rosemary, and lavender smell good. When a few drops of these essential oils are applied to the temple, they help relieve headaches, if you aren't allergic.

Another possible remedy is to stretch the muscles in your back or your neck, and yoga also offers relief in a few simple steps, as follows. Sit up straight in a comfortable position. Tilt your head to one side, and then use the opposite hand to gently increase the pressure. Breathe deeply while holding for a few seconds before switching sides.

Conventional care for migraines, usually medicine prescribed by a doctor, works better if accompanied by yoga practiced on a regular basis. A study showed that the frequency and intensity of debilitating episodes, as well as anxiety and depression, were reduced, when comparing a group of thirty who received conventional care only to a group of thirty who also received yoga therapy. Even doctors who practice yoga and believe in its restorative nature agree that further research needs to be conducted.

"A great wind is blowing,
and that gives you either
imagination or a headache."
– Catherine the Great

Help for Diabetes

If you are at risk for developing diabetes, there are numerous things you can do to delay or prevent the onset of the disease. You know what they are: manage your blood pressure; keep your weight in a healthy range; eat a balanced die; and exercise.

Yoga can be a part of your exercise regime. While it won't cure the condition, it helps control it, even eliminating the need for expensive medication.

Certain poses can help lower blood pressure, as well as blood sugar levels. Spinal twists and forward bends stimulate the pancreas and other organs and aid digestion, as well as keep you flexible. Still, never force yourself to do more than your body allows.

While research studies are often limited by small sample sizes, taken together studies suggest that yoga can have a significant role in better managing the condition.

"Diabetes taught me discipline."
– Sonia Sotomayor

Help for Indigestion

Who hasn't suffered from heart burn or bloating or been embarrassed by gas or flatulence. As we get older, our digestive system doesn't work as well as it used to, and these situations can become more common and frequent.

Certainly, there are foods, such as anything greasy, fried, or processed, that should be avoided. Medicines, either over-the-counter or prescribed, might provide relief.

Yoga can have a positive impact, either directly or indirectly. Through meditation, it reduces stress. Certain postures offer physical benefits by stimulating circulation, massaging the abdominal muscles, and balancing the metabolism. Breathing deeply throughout entire practice is always beneficial.

One study at the University of California, Los Angeles has shown that yoga, as well as walking, made a significant difference to adults with Irritable bowel syndrome and another, reported in the International Journal of Yoga, suggested that, along with medicine, yoga reduced the symptoms of those with gastro-esophageal reflux disease (GERD).

> **"You better cut the pizza in four pieces because I'm not hungry enough to eat six." – Yogi Berra**

Help for Memory Loss

The physical benefits of Have-A-Seat Yoga™ include flexibility and mobility, but it can prevent memory loss and improve cognitive abilities, as well.

Neuroscientists at the University of California, Los Angeles in 2016 measured the brain activity of twenty-five individuals over fifty-five years old, eleven of whom spent twenty minutes a day on memory exercises. The remainder of the group took a one-hour yoga class per week and carried out meditation, involving chanting, hand movements and visualization, for twenty minutes a day. After twelve weeks, everyone had enhanced their verbal skills, that is, their ability to remember names and lists of words. However, those who did yoga and meditation were more resilient and less anxious and showed significant improvement in their brain fitness, as indicated by MRI brain scans.

The study group was small, and it will need follow-up over a longer period of time.

However, it demonstrates the importance of exercise to mental health.

> "Life is all memory, except
> for the one present moment
> that goes by you so quickly
> you hardly catch it going."
> – Tennessee Williams

Help for Heart Disease

If you have been diagnosed with heart disease or suffered a heart attack, it's likely that you are worried, even depressed. Yoga can help. It not only helps manage stress, but also facilitates lower blood press, cholesterol, and glucose levels. Medical researchers at Johns Hopkins, the Harvard School of Public Health, and other institutions of higher learning reviewed research that showed this to be the case in study after study.

As examined in an article in the *Journal of the American College of Cardiology*, yoga combined with aerobic exercise, rather than yoga or exercise alone, has an even more positive impact on cardiovascular health.

> **"You wake up one day and suddenly realize that your youth is behind you, even though you're still young at heart."**
> **– Joni Mitchell**

Appendix

WHAT INSPIRES YOU?

T his is not the end. It's only the beginning. Whether or not you are keeping a journal, write down what inspires you. Tell us. Contact Kelly on breathtobalance.com. Tell someone you know. Inspire them.

— — — — — — — — — —

If you are an administrator or a certified instructor, please contact Kelly for information on how you can bring the Have-A-Seat Yoga™ program to your residents and students. She will be-happy to discuss how you can receive complimentary copies of *Have-A-Seat Yoga™ : Inspiration*, purchase the book at bulk discounts, or become a part of the Have-A-Seat Yoga™ team.

CPSIA information can be obtained
at www.ICGtesting.com
Printed in the USA
FSHW021546290120
66570FS